1

Table of Contents

PREVIEW 4

PANCREATIC CANCER DIET RECIPES 5

BREAKFAST 5

1. Apricot Chicken.. 5

2. Avocado Deviled Eggs... 7

3. Chickpea Pancakes with Jellyberry Grape Jam & Almond Butter 9

4. Chickpea Crepes with Spinach and Mushroom Pesto 12

5. Apricot Pecan Bars... 15

6. Bagel Avocado Toast with Salmon 17

7. Maple Walnut Granola 20

8. Mediterranean White Bean and Sorghum Salad........................... 22

9. Quinoa with Cauliflower and Broccoli 25

10. Cauliflower Osso Bucco 27

LUNCH... 29

11. Spring Stir Fry with Chicken... 29

12. Quinoa Risotto Primavera 31

13. Spinach and Goat Cheese Stuffed Portobellos........................... 33

14. Get Nutty Whole Grain Banana Bread 35

15. Cranberry-Apple Hazelnut Crumble 37

16. Layered Nachos Grandes 39

17. Almond Crusted Baked Chicken Tenders 42

18. Picnic Pasta Salad with Cotton Candy Grapes, Baby Spinach, and Feta 45

19. Spring Salad with Edamame, Cucumber, Snow Peas and Tofu Croutons 47

20. Pumpkin Mac and Cheese 49

DINNERS 52

21. Moroccan Chickpea Sorghum Bowl.................................. 52

22. Scrambled Turmeric Tofu with Greens.......................... 54

23. Fresh and Light Veggie Pad Thai.................................. 56

24. Tex-Mex Sorghum Chili... 59

25. Citrus Quinoa Avocado Salad 61

26. Vegan Tofu Lasagna 63

27. Rosemary Garlic Flatbread 65

28. Roasted Ratatouille Vegetable Dip 68

29. Easy Summer Lasagna 70

30. Walnut Tomato Sauce with Zucchini Lasagna Noodles 72

Pancreatic cancer is usually not found until advanced stages because it is hard to detect. Signs of pancreatic cancer include jaundice and weight loss. Risk factors include having diabetes and exposure to certain chemicals. Specific treatment depends on the size and location of the tumor, and whether or not it has spread to other areas of the body.

BREAKFAST

1. Apricot Chicken

Prep Time: 40

430 calories per serving

Ingredients

- 1 cup apricot jam or marmalade
- 2 tsp. garlic, minced
- 1 1/2 Tbsp. olive oil
- 1 Tbsp. soy sauce
- 2 tsp. Dijon mustard
- 1/2 small jalapeño, deseeded and minced (optional)
- 2 tsp. fresh ginger, grated
- 1/2 tsp. salt
- Black pepper, to taste
- 4 (6 oz.) boneless skinless chicken breasts, pounded thin with rolling pin or meat pounder
- 4 apricots, under-ripe, quartered and pitted*
- 1/2 red onion, sliced

Instructions

1. Preheat oven to 350 degrees F.

2. In medium bowl, mix jam, garlic, olive oil, soy sauce, mustard, jalapeño, ginger, salt and pepper, to taste.

3. Add chicken breasts and stir to coat.

4. Place apricots and onion slices on oiled baking sheet and then place chicken breast mixture on top, nestling apricots and onions around breasts.

5. Cook for 20 25 minutes, flipping halfway through. Chicken is done when a meat thermometer registers 165 degrees F.

Prep Time: 30

130 calories per serving

Ingredients

- 12 eggs
- 2 medium avocados, chopped
- 1 medium tomato, chopped
- 2 Tbsp. red onion, finely chopped
- 1 clove garlic, minced
- 1 Tbsp. cilantro, finely chopped
- 1 Tbsp. fresh lime juice
- 1/4 tsp salt
- Sprinkle of paprika
- 1/2 jalapeño pepper, minced (optional

Instructions

1. Hard boil eggs by placing eggs in an even layer in large pot covered by 2 inches of cold water. Heat pan on high and bring to rolling boil. Immediately turn off heat, cover pot with lid and let eggs sit on hot burner for 10 minutes.

2. Transfer eggs to bowl of ice water to cool; peel eggs.

3. Slice eggs lengthwise and scoop out yolks; place yolks in large mixing bowl.

4. Add avocados to yolks and mash with fork until completely mixed.

5. Add remaining ingredients, except paprika. Stir to combine.

6. Carefully scoop about 1 Tbsp. of mixture into each egg white half.

7. Sprinkle with paprika to garnish.

8. Top with jalapeño, if using.

Prep Time: 30

240 calories per serving

Ingredients

For the Jam:

- 2 cups purple grapes, cut in half
- 2 Tbsp. lemon juice
- 1 tsp. honey
- 1/4 tsp. ground cinnamon
- Pinch of salt. or to taste
- 1 tsp. cornstarch
- 1 Tbsp. water

For the Pancakes:

- 1 cup chickpea flour
- 2 tsp. baking powder
- 1/4 tsp. ground cinnamon
- Pinch of salt, or to taste
- 3/4 cup plain unsweetened almond milk
- 1 tsp. honey
- 1/2 tsp. vanilla extract

- Nonstick cooking spray
- 4 Tbsp. almond or peanut butter

Instructions

1. Place small saucepan over medium heat. Add grapes, lemon juice, honey, cinnamon and salt and stir to combine. Bring to low boil, lower heat, and simmer, uncovered, stirring occasionally, until grapes soften, about 8 minutes.

2. Place cornstarch and water in small bowl and whisk to combine. Stir into grape mixture and cook, stirring frequently, until thickened, 1 to 2 minutes. Set aside.

3. Meanwhile, place chickpea flour, baking powder, cinnamon and salt in medium-size bowl and whisk until well combined. Whisk in almond milk, honey and vanilla until well combined.

4. Spray a 10-inch nonstick skillet with nonstick cooking spray and heat over medium heat. Pour in 1/3 cup of batter and cook until golden on the bottom, 2 to 3 minutes. Adjust heat to medium-low if bottom browns too quickly. Flip and cook another 2 minutes. Repeat with cooking spray and remaining batter. Keep pancakes warm between batches.

5. To serve, spread 1 tablespoon almond butter evenly over each pancake. Top evenly with Jellyberry grape jam.

Prep time: 70 minute

170 calories per serving

Ingredients

Crepes:

- 1 cup chickpea flour
- 2 Tbsp. extra-virgin olive oil
- 1 tsp. finely chopped fresh rosemary
- 1/4 tsp. salt
- 1 cup water
- 2 tsp. soft buttery spread, if using skillet

Filling:

- 2 tsp. extra-virgin olive oil
- 1/4 cup finely chopped red onion
- 1/3 cup finely chopped red bell pepper
- 6 oz. cremini mushrooms, thinly sliced (about 2 cups)
- 1 box (5oz.) baby spinach
- 2 Tbsp. prepared pesto
- Salt and freshly ground black pepper, to taste

Instructions

1. In medium bowl, whisk chickpea flour, oil, rosemary and salt with 1 cup water until mixture is smooth. Let batter sit 20-30 minutes to thicken. Before cooking, stir to loosen any clumps.

2. For crepes, set non-stick pan over medium-high heat until drops of water flicked into pan ball up and bounce. With one hand, hold pan up at 45-degree angle. Pour ¼ cup batter near top of pan, rotating pan as you pour so batter flows into 6-7-inch round crepe. Cook until crepe is golden on bottom, 1-2 minutes. Using large spatula, flip and cook until crepe is lightly golden on bottom, about 30 seconds. Transfer crepe to large plate. Cover each crepe with wax paper.

3. If not filling crepes immediately, cool to room temperature and cover plate with plastic wrap. Hold crepes at room temperature for up to 8 hours, refrigerate for up to 24 hours.

4. For filling, in medium skillet heat oil over medium-high heat. Add onion and cook, stirring for 2 minutes. Add red peppers and cook, stirring, until onions are translucent, 5 minutes. Add mushrooms and cook, stirring occasionally, until mixture looks wet, 5-6 minutes. Add spinach, stirring to wilt leaves. Cook,

stirring often, until most of moisture has evaporated and filling is tender, 8 minutes.

5. If crepes have been made ahead, wrap them in foil and warm at 250 degree F for 20 minutes. To assemble crepes, in small bowl, mix pesto with 2 tbsp. warm water. Stir pesto into filling. Arrange a crepe on a plate. Spoon ⅙ filling over bottom half of each crepe, then gently fold crepe in half over filling. Repeat with remaining crepes and filling. If desired, garnish plate with some mesclun leaves and strawberries. Serve immediately.

Prep time: 65

190 calories per serving

Ingredients

- 3 cups quick cooking oats
- 1/2 cup pecans, chopped
- 3 cups unsweetened grain cereal (cheerios or shredded wheat)
- 2 cups dried apricots, chopped
- 1/4 cup whole-wheat flour
- 12 oz. silken tofu, drained
- 1 large egg
- 1/2 cup applesauce
- 1/2 cup canola oil
- 3/4 cup honey
- 1/2 tsp. salt
- 1 Tbsp. lemon zest, freshly grated
- 1 Tbsp. vanilla extract
- Canola oil cooking spray

Instructions

1. Preheat oven to 350 degrees F.

2. Spread oats and pecans on large (15x10 inch) baking dish. Bake until lightly brown and fragrant, 8 to 10 minutes.

3. Transfer to large mixing bowl and add cereal, apricots and flour; stir to combine.

4. Puree tofu, egg, applesauce, oil, honey, vanilla and lemon zest in a blender until smooth. Make a well in the center of the oat mixture and fold in the tofu mixture until combined. Coat 9x13 baking dish with cooking spray and spread the mixture uniformly in the dish.

5. Bake until firm in the center and golden brown, approximately 35 to 40 minutes. Let cool completely in the dish before cutting into bars with a sharp knife.

Prep time: 65

590 calories per serving

Ingredients

- 3 Tbsp. sesame seeds

- 3 Tbsp. poppy seeds

- 1 Tbsp. dried minced onion

- 2 tsp. dried minced garlic

- 1/2 tsp. coarse or flaked salt

- 1 egg white

- 2 Tbsp. cornstarch

- 4 (4-ounces each) wild Alaska salmon fillets, preferably cut from the thinner tail end

- 2 Tbsp. olive oil

- 2 whole grain bagels, halved and toasted

- 1 avocado, seeded, sliced, and scooped

- 2 small lemons, quartered

- Salt and pepper, to taste

- 8 slices tomato (4 if tomatoes are large)

- 4 slices red onion

- 4 tsp. capers (optional)

- 1 tsp. chopped parsley, for garnish

Instructions

1. In a bowl, stir together the sesame seeds, poppy seeds, dried onion, dried garlic and salt.

2. In a small bowl with a fork, stir the egg white and cornstarch together until smooth. Brush the skinless sides of the salmon fillets with the egg-white mixture. Spread the seeds on a plate. Press the skinless side of salmon fillets into the seeds to coat them.

3. In a large nonstick frying pan over medium heat, heat the oil. Cook the salmon, seed-side down, for 1 to 2 minutes, or until golden brown. The seeds brown quickly, so check after 1 minute. Turn and cook on the other side for 2 to 3 minutes, or until a thermometer inserted into the thickest part of the salmon should register at 125° F. The exact time will vary according to the thickness of the fillets. Transfer the cooked salmon to a plate and cover loosely with foil while you prepare the bagels. The salmon will continue to cook as it rests.

4. On a cutting board, spread the toasted bagel halves. Top with the avocado slices. Mash them with a fork or leave them in slices. Sprinkle with lemon juice, salt and pepper. Top each bagel half with 2 tomato slices.

5. Place the cooked salmon pieces on top of each bagel. Top with the onion slices, capers and parsley and serve with the remaining lemon wedges.

Prep time: 65

220 calories per serving

Ingredients

- Nonstick cooking spray
- 3 cups old fashioned oats
- 1/4 cup whole-wheat flour
- 1/4 cup chopped English walnuts
- 1/2 tsp. cinnamon
- Pinch of salt
- 1/3 cup maple syrup
- 1/3 cup canola oil
- 1 tsp. vanilla extract

Instructions

1. Preheat oven to 300 degrees F. Lightly coat a large baking sheet with cooking spray.
2. In large bowl, combine oats, flour, walnuts, cinnamon and salt. In separate bowl whisk together maple syrup, oil and vanilla. Add to oat mixture, stirring well to coat.
3. On large baking sheet, evenly spread mixture. Bake 30 minutes. Remove tray from oven and stir granola,

breaking up any lumps. Return to oven and bake an additional 20 minutes.

4. Remove from oven and allow granola to cool completely. Store in airtight container.

Prep Time: 55 minute

400 calories per serving

Ingredients

Sorghum:

- 3 cups water
- 1 cup whole grain sorghum, uncooked

Roasted Vegetables and White Beans:

- 2 medium carrots, sliced
- 1 small green bell pepper, sliced
- 1 small red onion, sliced
- 1 can (15.5 oz.) white beans, rinsed, drained
- 1 small head cauliflower, separated into small florets
- 1 1/2 Tbsp. extra virgin olive oil
- 1/2 lemon, juiced
- 1 tsp. dried oregano
- 1/2 tsp. garlic powder
- 2 Tbsp. fresh chopped parsley (or 1 tsp. dried)
- 1 Tbsp. fresh chopped rosemary (or 1 tsp. dried)
- 1/4 tsp. black pepper

- 1 Sea salt (as desired, optional)

Add-ons:

- 4 cups baby kale
- 1/2 lemon, sliced into 4 wedges
- 1/4 cup roasted pistachios

Instructions

1. In a medium saucepan, bring 3 cups of water to a boil. Add sorghum, cover, and simmer over medium for about 45 minutes, until just tender. Remove from burner. Drain any remaining liquid.
2. While sorghum is cooking, prepare roasted vegetables and white beans.
3. Preheat oven to 375 F.
4. On a baking sheet, arrange a thin layer in vertical sections of: carrots slices, green bell pepper slices, red onion slices, white beans, and cauliflower florets.
5. Drizzle oil and lemon juice evenly over the vegetables.
6. Sprinkle the vegetables evenly with: oregano, garlic powder, parsley, rosemary, black pepper, and sea salt (if desired).

7. Mix the seasonings into the vegetables with tongs (or your hands) to distribute well.

8. Place on top rack of the oven and roast for about 30 minutes, until golden brown and tender. Remove from the oven.

9. Prepare each salad: In each of four glass rectangular containers, arrange kale, and top with one-fourth of the cooked sorghum and one-fourth of the roasted vegetables and white beans. Garnish with roasted pistachios. Add a lemon wedge. Cover and refrigerate for up to 5 days.

10. To serve, squeeze lemon wedge over salad and enjoy!

Prep time: 50 minute

120 calories per serving

Ingredients

- 1 Tbsp. extra-virgin olive oil, divided
- 2 cups cauliflower florets
- 2 cups broccoli florets
- 1 medium green bell pepper, sliced into strips
- 1 medium red bell pepper, sliced into strips
- 1 cup chopped onion, divided
- 3 cloves garlic, minced
- 1 Tbsp. fresh thyme, chopped medium (1 tsp. dried may be substituted)
- 1 Tbsp. fresh oregano, chopped medium (1 tsp. dried may be substituted)
- 1 cup quinoa, well rinsed and drained
- 2 cups fat free, reduced-sodium vegetable broth
- Salt and freshly ground black pepper

Instructions

1. In skillet, heat 2 tsp. olive oil over medium-high heat. Add cauliflower, broccoli, peppers, ½ cup onion and garlic. Sauté 5 minutes until vegetables start to soften. Stir in herbs and sauté 2 minutes. Remove from stove top and set aside.

2. In strainer, place quinoa and rinse thoroughly with cold water. Using your hand, swish quinoa under running water for 2 minutes to remove bitter natural coating. Drain and set aside.

3. In medium saucepan, heat remaining teaspoon oil over medium-high heat. Add remaining onion. Sauté about 3 to 4 minutes. Add broth and quinoa. Increase heat to bring mixture to boil. Reduce heat to medium-low, cover, and simmer until quinoa is tender, about 20 minutes.

4. Gently stir in vegetable mixture and combine well with quinoa. Season with salt and pepper to taste. Serve.

Prep Time: 60 minute

210 calories per serving

Ingredients

- 1 lb fresh cauliflower head
- 1/4 cup white whole-wheat flour
- 1 Tbsp. olive oil
- 2 cloves garlic, minced
- 2 carrots, chopped
- 2 tsp. lemon zest
- 1 cup no salt added tomato paste
- 1 1/2 cups low sodium vegetable broth (may need more)
- Salt and black pepper, to taste

Instructions

1. Preheat oven to 350 degrees F.
2. Wash and slice cauliflower into "steaks."
3. Dredge cauliflower in flour (you may need to dip it in water briefly first to get the flour to stick).Place olive oil in large skillet and briefly brown the cauliflower steaks

on medium high heat until they are a rich golden color. Turn at least once during cooking to prevent burning and ensure steaks have a slight golden crust on both sides.

4. Push cauliflower to the side of the pan (or remove it to a plate if pan is too crowded) and add the garlic, carrots and lemon zest. Sauté for 3-5 minutes, stirring occasionally.

5. Add the tomato paste and broth and stir until blended. (If you removed the cauliflower from the pan in step 3, add it back to the pan at this time.)

6. Cover the pan and place in the 350 degree F oven to bake for approximately 45 minutes until the cauliflower is soft and the sauce is blended.

7. Adjust seasonings if needed. To serve, garnish with gremolata.

8. To make gremolata,: Using a small bowl, combine 4 cloves of finely minced garlic, 1/2 cup washed and finely chopped fresh parsley, and 1 Tbsp. lemon zest. Cover and refrigerate until ready to use.

11. Spring Stir Fry with Chicken

Prep Time: 40 minute

440 calories per serving

Ingredients

- 1 Tbsp. peanut oil
- 5 cloves garlic
- 1 tsp. grated fresh ginger
- 1/4 tsp. ground ginger
- 6 spring onions, chopped, including the green stems
- Salt, to taste
- 1 lb. chicken, boneless and skinless, cut into ½ -inch strips
- 1 large onion, chopped
- 1 cup chopped cabbage
- 1 medium red bell pepper, chopped
- 1 medium green bell pepper, chopped
- 2 Tbsp. reduced-sodium soy sauce
- 1 1/2 tsp. sugar (optional)
- 1 Tbsp. cornstarch

- 1/2 cup water
- 3 cups cooked brown rice

Instructions

1. In a wok or large skillet, heat oil over medium-high heat. When oil is almost smoking, add garlic, ginger, ground ginger, spring onions and salt to taste. Stir-fry for 2 minutes. Add chicken. Stir-fry an additional 3 to 4 minutes.
2. Add chopped onion and cabbage and cook, stirring occasionally, for about 5 minutes. Add peppers and cook for 2 minutes.
3. Mix soy sauce, sugar and cornstarch into water, then add to wok or skillet. Cook uncovered until sauce thickens. Serve over hot rice.

Prep Time: 45 minute

120 calories per serving

Ingredients

- 2.5 cups cauliflower florets cut into 1-inch pieces, stems well-trimmed
- 1 1/2 tbsp extra virgin olive oil
- 1/2 cup finely chopped onion
- 2 Tbsp. finely chopped shallot
- 2/3 cup quinoa, rinsed and drained
- 3 1/2 cups fat-free, reduced sodium chicken broth, divided
- 1/3 cup thinly sliced baby carrots
- 1/2 cup frozen peas
- 1/4 cup grated Parmesan cheese
- salt and freshly ground black pepper
- 1/3 cup chopped flat leaf parsley

Instructions

1. Place cauliflower in food processor. Pulse until cauliflower resembles crumbled feta, about 15-20

pulses; there should be 2 cups chopped cauliflower to set aside. Add leftovers to soup or salad.

2. In heavy, wide, large saucepan, heat oil over medium-high heat. Add onion and cook, stirring often, for 3 minutes. Add shallots and cook until golden, about 3 minutes, stirring occasionally. Add quinoa and cook, stirring constantly, until grain makes constant crackling, popping sound, about 5 minutes. Carefully add 2 cups broth, standing back as it will spatter. Cover, reduce heat and simmer quinoa for 10 minutes.

3. Add cauliflower, carrots and 1/2 cup hot broth and simmer, uncovered, for 5 minutes, stirring often. Add peas and enough broth to keep risotto soupy, about 1/4 cup. Cook 8-10 minutes, or until quinoa is al dente or to your taste and vegetables are tender-crisp, adding broth 1/4 cup at a time, as needed. Risotto is done when liquid is mostly absorbed and mixture is slightly wet, but not soupy. Off heat, stir in cheese and season to taste with salt and pepper. Garnish with parsley and serve. Leftover risotto keeps for 3 days, covered in refrigerator, and can be served at room temperature as a whole-grain salad.

Prep Time: 25 minute

240 calories per serving

Ingredients

- 4 large portobello mushroom caps
- 2 Tbsp. olive oil, divided
- 3 small shallots, chopped
- 3 cloves garlic, chopped
- 6 oil-packed sun-dried tomatoes, drained and chopped
- 5 cups raw baby spinach
- 1/4 tsp. black pepper
- 1 cup cherry tomatoes, quartered
- 1/4 cup grated Parmesan cheese, divided
- 4 oz. goat cheese sliced
- 1 Tbsp. balsamic vinegar, divided
- 8 basil leaves, thinly sliced

Instructions

1. Preheat oven to 400°F.
2. Using damp paper towel or cloth, gently wipe any dirt from portobello caps. Use small knife to slice off each stem at base of caps and discard.

3. Coat mushroom caps on each side using 1 Tbsp. olive oil. Place mushrooms gill-side up on a baking sheet and roast until they start to soften, about 10 minutes. While mushrooms are roasting, make the filling.

4. Heat large skillet over medium heat and add 1 Tbsp. olive oil until it begins to shimmer. Add shallots and garlic and sauté 1-2 minutes, until translucent.

5. Add sun-dried tomatoes and stir.

6. Add spinach and stir gently until spinach begins to wilt, about 1 minute. Add pepper.

7. Add cherry tomatoes and sauté for another minute. Remove pan from heat and set aside.

8. Remove mushrooms from oven and divide spinach mixture evenly among each portobello cap.

9. Top each cap with 1 Tbsp. Parmesan cheese and 1 oz. goat cheese. Broil mushroom caps an additional 1-2 minutes until cheese starts to melt.

10. Serve each cap topped with a drizzle of balsamic vinegar and basil.

Prep Time: 80 minute

221 calories per serving

Ingredients

- 3 ripe medium bananas, peeled, mashed
- 1/2 cup milk or soy milk, plain, unsweetened
- 1/4 cup vegetable oil
- 2 Tbsp. chia seeds
- 1 tsp. vanilla
- 1/4 cup brown sugar
- 1 1/4 cups whole-wheat flour
- 1 tsp. baking soda
- 1/2 tsp. baking powder
- 1/2 tsp. cinnamon
- Pinch salt (optional)
- 2 Tbsp. sunflower seeds
- 2 Tbsp. coconut, unsweetened, shredded
- 2 Tbsp. sliced almonds
- 3 Tbsp, pistachio nuts
- 3 Tbsp. chopped walnuts
- Nonstick cooking spray

Instructions

1. Preheat oven to 350 degrees F.

2. In mixing bowl, whip together bananas, soy milk, vegetable oil, chia seeds, vanilla and sugar for two minutes. For best results, use an electric mixer.

3. Stir in remaining ingredients, mixing only until well combined.

4. Spray loaf pan with nonstick cooking spray.

5. Pour batter into loaf pan and bake for about 65 minutes, until fork inserted in center comes out clean.

6. Remove, cool slightly before slicing.

Prep Time: 70 minute

240 calories per serving

Ingredients

Fruit Filling:

- 10 oz. fresh or frozen cranberries, unsweetened
- 3 medium apples, peeled, sliced
- 1 orange, zest and juice
- 1/2 cup brown sugar

Whole Grain Crumble Topping:

- 1 cup old-fashioned oats
- 1/3 cup whole-wheat flour
- 1/3 cup hazelnuts, coarsely chopped
- 1 tsp. cinnamon
- 1 tsp. cardamom
- 1/2 tsp. ground ginger
- Pinch salt (optional)
- 1/4 cup vegetable oil

Instructions

1. Preheat oven to 375 F.

2. Place cranberries and apples in 9-inch pie dish or baking pan. Add zest, orange juice and brown sugar. Toss well.

3. In small bowl, combine oats, flour, hazelnuts, cinnamon, cardamom, ginger and salt, if using. Stir in oil with fork to make a crumbly mixture.

4. Sprinkle crumb topping over cranberry-apple filling and bake uncovered for 45-55 minutes, until golden brown.

Prep Time: 30 minute

280 calories per serving

Ingredients

Salsa Fresca:

- 1 cup finely chopped ripe tomato, seeded
- 1/2 cup drained canned no-salt added diced tomatoes
- 1/2 cup finely chopped onion
- 1/2 cup cilantro, chopped
- 1 jalapeño or Serrano pepper, seeded and very finely chopped
- 1 tsp. fresh lime juice

Refried Black Beans:

- 2 tsp. canola oil
- 1 can (15 oz.) no-salt added black beans, rinsed and drained
- 1 tsp. ground cumin
- Cooking spray

Nachos:

- 24 Restaurant-style reduced-sodium tortilla chips
- 1/2 cup shredded Pepper Jack cheese
- 8 tsp. reduced-fat sour cream
- 8 cilantro leaves
- 1 large jalapeño pepper, sliced into thin rounds
- 4 (¼ -inch wide) avocado slices, halved crosswise
- 1/2 lime

Instructions

1. Preheat oven to 350 degrees F. Line baking sheet with baking parchment and set aside.
2. To make salsa fresca, in mixing bowl, use fork to combine fresh tomato, canned tomato, onion, cilantro, chile pepper, and lime juice. Season to taste with salt and pepper. There will be 2 cups salsa. Set aside.
3. To make refried beans, coat cast iron or other heavy medium skillet with cooking spray. Heat oil over medium-high heat. Add beans and cumin and ½ cup water. Using sturdy fork, mash beans until lumpy and a bit soft. Season to taste with salt. Set aside ½ cup, reserving remaining beans for another use.

4. To assemble nachos, arrange 8 tortilla chips on prepared baking sheet. Top each chip with 1 tbsp. refried black beans. Add ½ tbsp. cheese. Top with second tortilla chip. Sprinkle on ½ tbsp. cheese.

5. Bake chips until cheese melts, about 4 minutes.

6. Using wide spatula, transfer two stacked nachos to each of 4 plates. Spoon 1 tbsp. salsa fresca on top of melted cheese and top each nacho with a third tortilla chip. Top with another tbsp. salsa fresca, the sour cream, cilantro, jalapeño and avocado. Add a squirt of lime juice. Serve immediately.

Prep Time: 40 minute

320 calories per serving

Ingredients

Chicken Tenders:

- 1 1/4 cup almonds
- 1 tsp. garlic powder
- 1 tsp. smoked paprika
- 1 tsp. dried mustard
- 1 tsp. dried oregano
- 1 tsp. dried thyme
- 1 tsp. salt
- 1/2 tsp. black pepper
- 2 eggs beaten
- 2 lbs. thin-sliced chicken breast halves (cut in half) or chicken tenders

Greek Yogurt Ranch Dip:

- 1 cup nonfat Greek yogurt
- 1/3 cup cup buttermilk
- 1 Tbsp. dried parsley

- 2 tsp. garlic powder

- 2 tsp. onion powder

- 1/8 tsp. cayenne pepper

- 1/8 tsp. ground black pepper

- 1/2 tsp. salt

- 2 eggs, beaten

- 1 tsp. Dijon mustard

- 1 tsp. lemon juice

- 1 Tbsp. fresh chives, finely chopped

- Fresh chives for garnish

Greek Yogurt Honey Mustard:

- 1/2 cup nonfat Greek yogurt

- 1 Tbsp. honey

- 1 Tbsp. yellow mustard

- 2 Tbsp. Dijon mustard

- 1/8 tsp. salt

Instructions

1. Preheat oven to 375 degrees.

2. In food processor, pulse almonds until finely ground
   into an almond meal.

3. Mix the almond meal together with garlic, paprika, dried mustard, oregano, thyme, salt and pepper.

4. Dredge each piece of chicken in egg and coat with almond spice mixture.

5. Place pieces on lightly greased cookie sheet.

6. Bake for 20-25 minutes, until golden.

7. For the Greek yogurt ranch dip, stir together all ingredients in a medium bowl, except for chives. Garnish with fresh chives and serve chilled.

8. For the honey mustard, mix all ingredients together and serve chilled.

Prep Time: 35 minute

230 calories per serving

Ingredients

For the Vinaigrette:

- 1/4 cup extra-virgin olive oil
- 2 Tbsp. lemon juice
- 2 tsp. Dijon mustard
- 1 tsp. champagne vinegar (or any other white vinegar)
- 1 small garlic clove, minced
- 1 tsp. honey or maple syrup
- Kosher salt, to taste
- Freshly ground black pepper, to taste

For the Pasta Salad:

- 8 oz. whole-wheat orzo pasta
- 1 1/2 cups green grapes, halved
- 1 small red bell pepper, cut into ¾-inch dice (about 1 cup)
- 1 cup packed baby spinach, roughly chopped

- 1/2 cup mint leaves, roughly chopped
- 1/3 cup diced red onion (cut into 1/4 inch dice)
- 1/3 cup pitted Kalamata olives, cut in half
- 1/3 cup crumbled feta cheese
- 2 Tbsp. roasted pumpkin seeds or sunflower seeds

Instructions

1. Place olive oil, lemon juice, mustard, vinegar, garlic and honey in small container with a tight-fitting lid and shake until well combined. Season with salt and pepper, to taste. Set aside.
2. Meanwhile, cook pasta according to package directions. Drain in colander when done, and rinse under cold water to cool.
3. Place pasta in large bowl. Stir in grapes, bell pepper, spinach, mint, onion, olives, feta and pumpkin seeds until well combined.
4. Add half the vinaigrette and stir well until all ingredients are well coated. Season with additional salt and pepper, to taste. Add remaining vinaigrette, if needed. (If making ahead and storing for several hours or overnight in refrigerator, stir in remaining vinaigrette before serving, if needed.)

Prep Time: 50 minute

260 calories per serving

Ingredients

- 1 block (14 oz.) firm tofu
- 1 Tbsp. sesame oil
- 1 Tbsp. low-sodium soy sauce
- 1 Tbsp. cornstarch
- 1 tsp. ground ginger
- 1 tsp. garlic powder
- pre-washed salad greens (about 5 oz.)
- 2 cups snow pea pods, trimmed and sliced on diagonal into 3/4-inch pieces
- 1 cup frozen shelled edamame, cooked according to package directions
- 1 English cucumber (4 in.), sliced in half lengthwise and cut into thin half-moons
- 1/4 cup loosely packed mint leaves, roughly chopped, or more to taste
- 1/4 cup sesame ginger salad dressing, or more to taste

Instructions

1. Preheat oven to 400 degrees F. Line a large, rimmed baking sheet with parchment paper and set aside. (If you don't have parchment paper, spray baking sheet with nonstick cooking spray.)

2. Place tofu in a colander and drain water. Wrap tofu in a few layers of paper towels and transfer to a cutting board. Press block under a baking sheet to squeeze out excess water. Stack something heavy on top such as a few cans of beans or a kettle filled with water. Let drain, about 20 minutes.

3. Remove paper towels. Cut tofu into forty-eight 3/4-inch cubes.

4. Meanwhile, in large bowl, whisk together sesame oil, soy sauce, cornstarch, ginger and garlic powder. Add tofu cubes and toss gently until well coated.

5. Transfer tofu to prepared baking sheet. Bake until golden, about 20 minutes. Turn cubes halfway through to ensure even baking.

6. Set out 4 dinner-size salad bowls. Fill each with salad greens, snow peas, edamame, cucumber, mint, dressing and tofu croutons. (Assemble in large bowl or on platter if you prefer serving family style.)

Prep Time: 30 minute

260 calories per serving

Ingredients

- Canola oil cooking spray
- 1/2 cup panko bread crumbs
- 1/3 cup grated Parmesan cheese
- 8 oz. whole-wheat pasta
- 1 cup low-fat (1%) milk
- 1 Tbsp. unsalted butter
- 1 Tbsp. all-purpose flour
- 1 1/2 cups (2 1/2 oz.) sharp light (50 percent) Cheddar cheese
- 1 cup canned unsweetened pumpkin
- 1/2 tsp. mustard powder
- 1/4 tsp. ground black pepper
- Pinch of cayenne pepper
- 1/8 tsp. ground nutmeg, optional

Instructions

1. Preheat oven to 375 degrees F. Coat 6 cup baking dish with cooking spray and set aside.

2. In a separate bowl mix together breadcrumbs and Parmesan cheese and toss to combine. Set mixture aside.

3. In large pot, boil 4 quarts of water. Add pasta and cook for 10 minutes, until slightly al dente. Drain in colander, and set aside.

4. While pasta is cooking, heat milk in microwave or small saucepan, until it steams, and set aside.

5. In large saucepan, melt butter over medium heat. Whisk in flour and cook for 1 minute, whisking slowly. Remove from heat and gradually add milk while whisking to avoid lumps. Return pot to medium-high heat and simmer sauce until it thickens to consistency of stirred yogurt, about 3 minutes.

6. Add Cheddar cheese, pumpkin, mustard, black and cayenne peppers and nutmeg (optional), and stir until cheese melts completely.

7. Mix in cooked pasta to cheese mixture.

8. Spread mac and cheese in prepared baking dish and sprinkle with breadcrumb and parmesan cheese mixture over top.

9. Bake 15-20 minutes or until breadcrumbs are crisp and golden brown. Serve immediately.

21. Moroccan Chickpea Sorghum Bowl

Prep Time: 60 minute

410 calories per serving

Ingredients

- 2 cups cooked whole grain sorghum
- 1 medium red onion, sliced into thin wedges
- 1 medium red bell pepper, sliced into thin strips
- 3 small carrots (red, purple, orange, yellow, or white), sliced
- 8 ounces Brussels sprouts, sliced in half vertically
- 1 15-ounce can chickpeas, rinsed, drained
- 2 Tbsp. extra virgin olive oil
- 1/4 cup fresh lemon juice
- 1 1/2 Tbsp. ras el hanout (Moroccan spice blend, see directions below)
- 2 garlic cloves, minced
- Pinch salt (optional)
- 2 cups chopped greens (i.e., kale, spinach, arugula leaves)
- 12 black olives (i.e., Kalamata, Picholine, Nicoise), rinsed, drained

Instructions

1. Cook sorghum according to package directions.

2. While sorghum is cooking, preheat oven to 375 F.

3. Arrange rows of sliced red onions, sliced red bell pepper, sliced carrots, halved Brussels sprouts, and chickpeas on a baking sheet (see picture).

4. Make the vinaigrette by whisking together olive oil, lemon juice, ras el hanout, garlic, and salt (optional) in a small dish.

5. Drizzle the vinaigrette evenly over the vegetables and chickpeas in the baking sheet.

6. Place on the top rack of the oven and roast for about 45 minutes, until vegetables are tender and golden brown.

7. Remove vegetables from oven.

8. To make each large individual bowl (makes 4 bowls): In each bowl, arrange 1/2 cup cooked sorghum on one side, and 1/2 cup greens on the other side. On each bowl, arrange on top of the sorghum and greens the following: 1/4 of the onions, 1/4 of the bell pepper, 1/4 of the carrots, 1/4 of the Brussels sprouts, 1/4 of the chickpeas, and 3 black olives.

9. Serve immediately.

Prep Time: 20 minute

152 calories per serving

Ingredients

- 1 14-oz. package extra- firm tofu
- 2 Tbsp. nutritional yeast
- 2 tsp. turmeric
- 1/4 tsp. smoked paprika
- 1/4 tsp. black pepper
- Pinch sea salt (optional)
- 2 Tbsp. plain, unsweetened soymilk
- 1 Tbsp. extra-virgin olive oil
- 2 green onions, sliced
- 2 cloves garlic, minced
- 6 oz. (about 2 1/4 cups) sliced mushrooms
- 2 cups loosely packed chopped greens (e.g., mustard, collard, spinach, kale)
- 1/4 cup sun-dried tomatoes, chopped

Instructions

1. Remove tofu from package and press it by wrapping it in paper towels and placing it between two plates with something heavy on top for 5 minutes, to allow extra liquid to drain off tofu.
2. Place tofu in bowl and break apart with your hands to achieve a crumbly texture. Mix in nutritional yeast, turmeric, smoked paprika, black pepper, salt (optional) and soymilk. Set aside.
3. Heat olive oil in skillet and sauté green onions, garlic and mushrooms for about 5 minutes.
4. Add crumbled tofu, chopped greens and sun-dried tomatoes and sauté just until greens start to wilt (about 2 minutes).
5. Serve immediately.

Prep Time: 45 minute

480 calories per serving

Ingredients

Pad Thai

- 8 ounces dried wide, flat rice noodles (preferably brown rice noodles)
- 1 Tbsp. olive, sesame, or canola oil (divided)
- 8 ounces extra firm tofu, drained and cut into ½ inch cubes
- 2 large eggs
- 1/2 yellow onion, chopped
- 3 cloves garlic, minced
- 1 head of broccoli, cut into small florets
- 1 zucchini, spiralized (or sliced into thin, long strips)
- 1 cup snap peas
- 2 carrots, grated
- 1 cup mung bean sprouts
- 1/4 cup fresh basil, chopped
- 1/4 cup fresh cilantro, chopped
- Crushed red pepper, to taste

Sauce

- 1 Tbsp. fish sauce
- 2 Tbsp. rice vinegar
- 1 Tbsp. reduced sodium soy sauce or tamari (gluten-free)
- 1 Tbsp. honey (or sub another sweetener)
- 1/4 cup lime juice (juice of 1-2 limes)

Garnishes

- 2 Tbsp. peanuts, chopped
- Lime wedges

Instructions

1. Prepare the sauce by whisking together all the sauce ingredients in a small bowl and set aside.
2. Next, prepare the noodles according to package instructions. For most rice noodles: bring a pot of water to a boil, remove from heat and let the noodles soak in the hot water until just al dente (about 10 minutes). Drain and set noodles aside.
3. Heat 1/2 of the oil over medium-high heat.

4. Sauté tofu about 3 minutes, or until just getting golden brown. Rotate the pieces to get a golden color on all sides. Move it to the edge of the pan.

5. Crack eggs into the pan, sauté with spatula to break yolk and scramble until just cooked through (about 1 min). Set the egg and tofu aside on a plate for a later step.

6. Add the remaining oil to the pan and add the onion and garlic. Sauté 1-2 minutes, or until just translucent. Optional: add a pinch of red chili flakes for extra heat.

7. Sauté the rest of your vegetables until they are just fork-tender and still bright in color, about 3 minutes.

8. Add the noodles, sauce, and tofu/egg mixture to the pan. Gently mix everything together so the flavors combine and the noodles can soak up the sauce. Add most of the herbs and bean sprouts (reserve a handful for garnish).

9. Serve with a topping of fresh herbs, the remaining bean sprouts, lime wedges, and a sprinkle of peanuts.

Prep Time: 115 minute

280 calories per serving

Ingredients

- 2 cups dried black beans
- 1 1/2 cups dried whole grain sorghum
- 4 cups water
- 4 cups vegetable broth, low sodium
- 3 stalks celery, diced
- 1 large onion, diced
- 3 cloves garlic, minced
- 1 green bell pepper, diced
- 1 cup yellow corn, frozen or canned, drained
- 1 14.5-ounce can fire-roasted, crushed tomatoes with juice
- 2 Tbsp. tomato paste
- 3 Tbsp. Mexican seasoning blend*
- Salt to taste (optional)

Instructions

1. Place beans in a large pot, cover with water and soak
    overnight.

2. The next day, discard the water, and add 4 cups fresh
    water and 4 cups vegetable broth. Add dried sorghum,
    stir well, cover and simmer over medium-low heat for
    45 minutes, stirring occasionally.

3. Add celery, onion, garlic, pepper, corn, tomatoes,
    tomato paste, and Mexican seasoning blend. Stir well to
    combine. Cover and simmer for an additional 45
    minutes, stirring occasionally, until beans, sorghum,
    and vegetables are tender. May need to add additional
    water lost to evaporation. Should make a thick stew-like
    texture.

4. Serve in bowls and garnish as desired with tortilla
    chips, fresh avocado slices, green onion slices, chopped
    fresh cilantro, and chopped fresh tomatoes.

Prep Time: 20 minute

390 calories per serving

Ingredients

- 1/2 cup cucumber, diced
- 1 cup cherry tomatoes, cut in half
- 2 small cloves garlic, minced
- 1/4 cup red onion, chopped
- 1 bunch cilantro
- 2 cups spinach, thinly sliced
- 1 15.5 oz can no salt added garbanzo beans (drained and rinsed)
- 1 cup cooked and cooled quinoa
- 2 medium avocados, diced

For the dressing:

- Juice of 2 lemons
- Zest of 1 lemon
- 2 tsp. Dijon mustard
- 1 Tbsp. olive oil
- 1 tsp. honey
- 1/2 tsp. ground cumin

- Dash of cayenne pepper (optional)
- Salt and pepper, to taste

Instructions

1. Place all salad ingredients in a bowl.
2. Whisk all dressing ingredients together in a separate bowl.
3. Drizzle dressing over salad mixture and gently toss ingredients together until dressing is incorporated throughout.

Prep Time: 20 minutes

Cooking Time: 30 minutes

Serving: 8

Ingredients

- 2tbspolive oil
- 1/2tspsalt
- 1tspItalian seasoning
- 16ozextra firm tofu
- 2clovesgarlic (or 1 tsp powdered garlic)
- 1tbspnutritional yeast
- 10ozfrozen kale (or spinach, collards), defrosted, water extracted
- 1packagelasagna noodles
- 16oztomato sauce

Instructions

1. Preheat oven to 350°.
2. Drain the tofu and pat dry with paper towels.
3. Crumble into the bowl of a food processor or high-speed blender.

4. Add Italian seasoning, garlic and nutritional yeast.

5. Process on high until smooth and "ricotta-like".

6. Add the defrosted kale to the blended tofu mixture.

7. Cook lasagna noodles according to package directions until al dente. Drain and cool.

8. Pour about 1/2 cup pasta sauce into the bottom of a 9x13 inch baking or lasagna pan.

9. Layer noodles with tofu mixture and a few spoonfuls of sauce until you reach three layers.

10. Smother with remaining tomato sauce.

11. Bake for approximately 30 minutes until sauce is bubbly and lasagna is heated through.

Prep Time: 100 minute

180 calories per serving

Ingredients

- 2 cups chickpea flour
- 3/4 cup sorghum flour
- 1/4 cup golden flaxseed
- 1/4 cup lemon juice
- 1 small head of garlic
- 2 cups water
- 1 tsp. salt
- 1/2 tsp. grated lemon zest
- 4-5 sprigs of fresh rosemary, chopped (or 1 Tbsp dried)
- 1 Tbsp. olive oil, divided

Instructions

1. Preheat oven to 450 degrees F.

2. Slice off the top of the garlic head to expose the garlic cloves, wrap in foil and roast in the oven for about 30 minutes.

3. In a large bowl, mix flours, flaxseed, salt, zest, salt, and rosemary.

4. Add lemon juice and water and whisk to combine. The batter should be thick but not stiff; do not overmix (a few small lumps are fine).

5. If possible, let the mix sit for at least 30 minutes (the longer the better).

6. Remove garlic from oven when cloves are fork-soft and squeeze out the cloves. Roughly chop them (large pieces are fine) and stir them into the batter.

7. 10 minutes before you are ready to cook the flatbread, drizzle 1 Tbsp olive oil in your 12-inch skillet and set it in the oven to heat up.

8. Add about 1/2 - 1/3 of the batter to the pan (depending on how thick you want your flatbread) and tilt to coat evenly.

9. Place the pan in the oven to cook the flatbread for 10-15 minutes, or until you can easily lift it from the pan with a spatula and the bottom is getting golden brown.

10. Turn the oven to broil and broil for 2-3 minutes, or just until the top starts to brown.

11. Remove from oven, slide onto a cutting board, and slice into wedges.

12. Repeat with the 2nd batch of the batter

Prep Time: 55 minute

40 calories per serving

Ingredients

- 1 pound eggplant, peeled and cut into 1-inch pieces
- 12 ounces yellow summer squash, cut into 1-inch pieces
- 2 red bell peppers, stemmed, seeded and cut into 1-inch pieces
- 12 ounces cherry tomatoes
- 1 medium onion, peeled, cut into 1-inch pieces
- 3 garlic cloves, coarsely chopped
- 1/4 cup extra-virgin olive oil
- 1/2 tsp. salt
- freshly ground pepper, to taste
- 1/4 cup minced fresh basil
- 2 tsp. lemon juice
- 1/2 tsp. salt
- Freshly ground pepper, to taste
- 1/8 tsp. cayenne pepper (optional, to taste)

Instructions

1. Adjust oven rack to middle position and heat oven to 450 degrees F. Toss eggplant, squash, bell peppers, tomatoes, onion, garlic, oil, salt and pepper together on heavy rimmed baking sheet and spread into an even layer. Roast until vegetables are slightly softened and roasted, about 30 minutes, stirring halfway through roasting.

2. Remove baking sheet from oven and let rest until cool enough to handle. Transfer vegetables and pan juices into food processor. Add minced basil, lemon juice and cayenne pepper (if using). Blend until smooth.

3. Serve with whole-grain tortilla chips, pretzels or as a non-dairy topping for whole-wheat bagels or sandwiches.

Prep Time: 110 minute

360 calories per serving

Ingredients

- 2 eggplants (about 3 lbs.), quartered lengthwise
- 6 medium zucchini (about 3 lbs.)
- Canola oil cooking spray
- 15 oz. low-fat ricotta or low-fat cottage cheese (or a combination of both)
- 2 eggs
- 1/2 cup grated Parmesan cheese
- 1/2 tsp. ground nutmeg
- 1/2 tsp. garlic powder
- 4 cups low-sodium tomato sauce
- 1 lb. whole-wheat, no-boil lasagna noodles
- 3 cups part-skim mozzarella cheese

Instructions

1. Preheat oven to 450 degrees F. Grease a 13 x 9 x 2-inch baking pan, set aside.
2. Slice the eggplant and zucchini in ½ -inch slices. Layer on two baking sheets and coat both sides of the

vegetables with cooking spray. Roast for about 40 minutes.

3. Reduce the oven temperature to 375 degrees F.

4. Meanwhile, in a medium bowl, mix together the ricotta and/or cottage cheeses, eggs, Parmesan, nutmeg and garlic powder.

5. To assemble: spread a thin layer of sauce over the bottom of the prepared pan. Cover with a layer of pasta. Spread ⅓ of the ricotta mixture on top of pasta. Sprinkle ¼ of the mozzarella over the ricotta. Spoon ⅓ of the roasted vegetables on top. Top with ½ cup of tomato sauce and continue the assembly as directed until you have 4 layers of pasta and 3 layers of filling. Spread the remaining sauce on top and sprinkle with the remaining mozzarella cheese.

6. Cover the pan with aluminum foil and bake for 30 minutes. Uncover and continue to bake until golden and bubbly, about 15 minutes more. Let stand for 15 minutes before serving.

Prep Time: 85 minute

282 calories per serving

Ingredients

Zucchini "Lasagna Noodles":

- 4 small zucchini squash

- Walnut Tomato Sauce

- 1 Tbsp. extra-virgin olive oil

- 1 medium onion, finely diced

- 3 cloves garlic, minced

- 2 stalks celery, finely chopped

- 5 ounces (about 2 cups) mushrooms, thinly sliced

- 1 32-ounce jar marinara sauce

- 2 Tbsp. tomato paste

- 1 Tbsp. soy sauce

- 1/2 cup red wine*

- 1 Tbsp. Italian seasoning blend

- 1/2 tsp. black pepper

- 1/4 tsp. salt (optional)

- 1 1/2 cups ground walnuts, divided

- Nonstick cooking spray

Filling

- 1 cup shredded plant-based cheese

Garnish

- 2 Tbsp. chopped Italian parsley

Instructions

1. Slice zucchini horizontally into long, thin slices (about 5 horizontal slices per squash). Place on paper towels and set aside (to soak up extra moisture).

2. Place a Dutch oven or large saucepan on medium heat and add olive oil.

3. Add onion, garlic and celery, and sauté for 3 minutes, stirring frequently.

4. Add mushrooms and sauté for an additional 2 minutes.

5. Add marinara sauce, tomato paste, soy sauce, red wine, Italian seasoning, black pepper and salt (if using). Stir well and cover. Simmer over medium heat for 10-15

minutes, stirring occasionally, until thickened and vegetables are tender.

6. Measure out 1 1/4 cups ground walnuts (may chop in a food processor or high-powered blender; should resemble consistency of course grains of sand, but should not be overly processed to a flour texture), reserving remaining ¼ cup ground walnuts for topping. Add the 1 1/4 cups ground walnuts to the sauce, and heat for 2 minutes.

7. Preheat oven to 350 degrees F.

8. Spray a 13x9-inch baking dish with nonstick cooking spray. Place one-third (6-7 slices) of the zucchini slices on the bottom of the dish. Layer with one-third of the walnut tomato sauce. Sprinkle with 1/3 cup of the shredded cheese. Repeat layers two more times, for a total of three layers of zucchini, walnut tomato sauce and cheese.

9. Place baking dish in the oven uncovered and bake for 40 minutes.

10. Sprinkle remaining 1/4 cup ground walnuts over top of lasagna and set oven to broiler setting. Broil for 2 minutes, until golden brown.

11. Remove from oven, garnish with fresh chopped parsley, slice into squares and serve immediately